THE 9 BEST EXERCISES THAT LOSES BODY WEIGHT AND BELLY FATS FASTER.

SECRETS TO HEALTHY LIVING.

OBAMA BRANDSON.

TABLE OF CONTENTS

INTRODUCTION

The need to be in good health and physically fits cannot be overemphasized. According to experts, most drugs and supplements are the causes of cancer, hence, exercise is the best anti-depressant in the world that burns fats faster and it is free. Studies have shown that people accumulate fats in their body and become obese because of what they eat. Hence, it is imperative to know how exercise contributes to weight loss. In a recent research, 23% of

Americans both young and adults are obese; this is either they are hereditary or gain fats through eating of junks foods and this is worrisome because the obese falls sick easily, at times they are bullied in schools, colleges and even in market places. Hence, there is need to live a healthy life, cut down on junk foods, smoking and alcohol intake, exercise regularly and eat balanced diet.

THE BENEFITS OF EXERCISING THE BODY?

The health benefits of exercises daily are as follows:-

1. Exercises increase your chances of living longer. Research shows that physical activity can reduce your risk of dying early from the leading causes of death, like heart related diseases and breasts, colon, lungs, uterus or cervical cancer.

2.   Exercise reduces risk of falling. For older adults, studies show that doing balance and muscle strengthening activities helps to reduce the risk of falling.

3.   Exercise makes the body glow and radiant. A daily exercise along with diet plays an important role by controlling the weight of the body and preventing obesity.

4.   It strengthens the bones and muscles also improve the ability to do work. Regular exercises can also

help teenagers to build strong bones. With age, it can also slow the loss of bone density. During muscle strengthening, it can help you to maintain or increase strength of the muscle.

5. During exercise, the body releases chemicals that improves your mood and make you feel more relaxed. This helps you to overcome depression and reduces stress.

6. Regular exercises improve mental health, keep your thinking,

learning and analytical skills sharper as you age, it also stimulates your body to release proteins and other chemicals that improve the structure and function of your brain.

7. It keeps the body temperature at a normal state and helps your body manage blood sugar and insulin levels. Study has shown that exercise can lower your sugar level and help your insulin work well. This reduces the risk of type 2 diabetes and metabolic syndrome. For those that already have one of these

diseases, exercise can help them to manage it.

9 BEST EXERCISES THAT LOSES BODY WEIGHT AND BELLY FATS FASTER ARE:-

1. RUNNING OR JOGGING

Running or jogging are great exercises that help you to lose weight faster within a week. Although they look similar, the major difference is that running has a faster pace in terms of kilometer per hour than jogging. Studies have shown that a person that run can burn up to 360 calories in less than 60 minutes while someone jogging can only burn approximately 250 to 280 calories.

Notes, running or jogging burns belly and other fats that wraps around the heart that can cause diabetes and other chronic diseases. Running and jogging are good exercises that can be carried out anywhere for a faster weight loss.

2. WEIGHT TRAINING

People looking to lose weight faster uses weight training. Weight training helps to build stamina and promote muscle growth that keeps you physically fit and healthy. Research have shown that your body continues to burn calories many hours after a weight-training workout, compare to aerobic exercise.

3. WALKING AROUND.

One of the best exercises for weight loss and losing belly fat speedily is to walk a mile at least three to four times in a week.

It is the easiest and most convenient way to start exercising without feeling stressed. This type of exercise does not involve cost of buying training equipments and hiring of instructor. Walking can be done anytime either indoor (around the house, taking the stairs instead of using lift etc.) or outdoor by walking with your dog.

4. SWIMMING

Another way to lose weight and have a good body posture is by engaging in swimming.

Swimming as an exercise is recommended to only experience swimmers. To undergo swimming you need an instructor that will guide you through.

Research has shown that swimmers that are adequately train can compete under any condition. Remember, the faster you swim, the faster the numbers of calories burnt. This implies that fat burns faster when the under listed methods: - breaststroke, butterfly, backstroke, and freestyle are applied during swimming.

Swimming has many benefits, one of which is stable blood pressure.

5. CYCLING.

Cycling is one of the exercises that help you to lose weight; burns belly fat and improve your fitness. During cycling, blood circulates to all parts of the body faster, this helps to lower the risk of having heart attack, cancer etc.

Generally, cycling is known to be an outdoor exercise, but with the advent of modern day's technology, gyms and fitness centers have stationary bikes that allow you to cycle indoors.

Research have shown that regular cycling can increase your insulin sensitivity and does not stress your joints, therefore, it is recommended for adults and teenagers who wishes to lose weight and stay fit.

6. YOGA.

Before now, yoga was not known to be one of the exercises that can burn fat faster but through recent researches, it has become more popular. Interestingly, yoga is seen as an 'entertaining' exercise. Yoga has proven to have burn more calories and reduces stress. It also improves the general well being of the body both physically and mentally.

Aside from patronizing fitness centers for yoga exercise, you can pay for instructor and be guided properly at the comfort of your home. Note, the purpose is to achieve result which is weight loss.

7. PILATES.

Pilates is one of the exercises that may help you lose weight. Although it does not burns calories faster like running and jogging but it is best enjoyed over time.

To do Pilates, as first timer you need a fitness instructor at home or you join the fitness centers.

In recent times, studies have shown that Pilates exercise can improve the strength and general well being of the body. Apart from weight loss, it also lowers back pains, reduces waist and belly fats within 4 weeks.

8. INTERVAL TRAINING

Interval training is one of the ways that burn calories faster.

In a recent research, 10 active men found that interval training burned 30–35% more calories per minute than other types of exercises, including running, jogging, weight training and cycling.

It is recommended by experts that interval training should be incorporated in your daily routine for a faster result because of its effectiveness in burning belly fats.

9. SEX

According to experts, sex is one of the safest exercises that burns belly fat and calories faster. It is recommended that having sex 5- 6 times in a week lowers the risk of having prostate cancer and erectile dysfunction in men. In women, exercise increases sexual arousal.

In a recent study, a 150-pound person burns 105 calories within 25 minutes during sex.

Many other exercises can help boost your weight loss efforts but choosing sex as best exercise is fun and does not involve joints pains. During sexual intercourse, hitting or banging harder burns more calories. The benefits of having sex are: - it maintains normal blood pressure, keeps headache and mood swing away, controls blood circulation from the heart to every part of the body and makes you happy all day.

You can agree with me that the importance of sex cannot be ruled out in this context because it is a form of exercise that helps to strengthen the pelvic or abdominal region of the body.

HOW MUCH WEIGHT CAN YOU LOSE FROM EXERCISING?

How much weight you lose from exercising depends on the following factors:

• Starting weight: People with a higher starting weight typically have a higher basal metabolic rate. This is the amount of calories your body burns when exercising life-preserving functions. This means you will burn more calories during exercise and rest.

- **Age:** Older people tend to carry more fat mass and less muscle mass, which reduces your metabolic rate. A lower basal metabolic rate can make it more difficult to lose weight.

- **Gender:** Women tend to have a greater fat-to-muscle ratio than men, which can affect their basal metabolic rate. Researches shown that men loses weight faster than women, even if they eat the same amount of calories.

- **Diet:** Weight loss occurs when you burn more calories than what you consume. Thus, low calories are essential to losing weight.

- **Sleep:** Studies have found that a lack of sleep may slow the rate at which you lose weight and even increases your cravings for high calorie foods.

CONCLUSIONS

Generally, exercise has been known to be the best way to lose weight and burn belly fat without surgery. It is also good for your heart, helps to build stamina and main good posture of the body. Unfortunately, people go for supplements as an alternative. However, care must be taken because trying to lose weight faster can have negative health consequences. Studies have shown that obese that are hereditary and people with severe medical conditions must be cautious while exercising. For example, it can result in joint pains, malnutrition, dehydration, irregular periods, fatigue etc.

It is advisable in trying to lose weight and burn belly fat, consult your doctor.

In summary, things to know when exercising for weight loss are:-

From all the types of exercises for weight loss highlighted above, it is not a must that you engage in all of them, rather chose what will best work for you.

Alternatively, the best bet is to focus more on healthy lifestyles that will aid general weight loss, while also benefiting your health in a number of other positive ways.

Combining exercise with a healthy diet is the ideal way to lose weight, rather than depending on calorie restriction alone. However, when engaging in intense exercises, ensure you are eating enough calories to keep your energy levels up.

Moreover, focus on the intensity of the exercise you are doing, rather than the number of calories you are burning.

Finally, by focusing on exercises you enjoy, you will be less concerned with how many calories you are actually burning during the activities.